Olivia McNeal

LIVE BETTER

with

A-to-Z

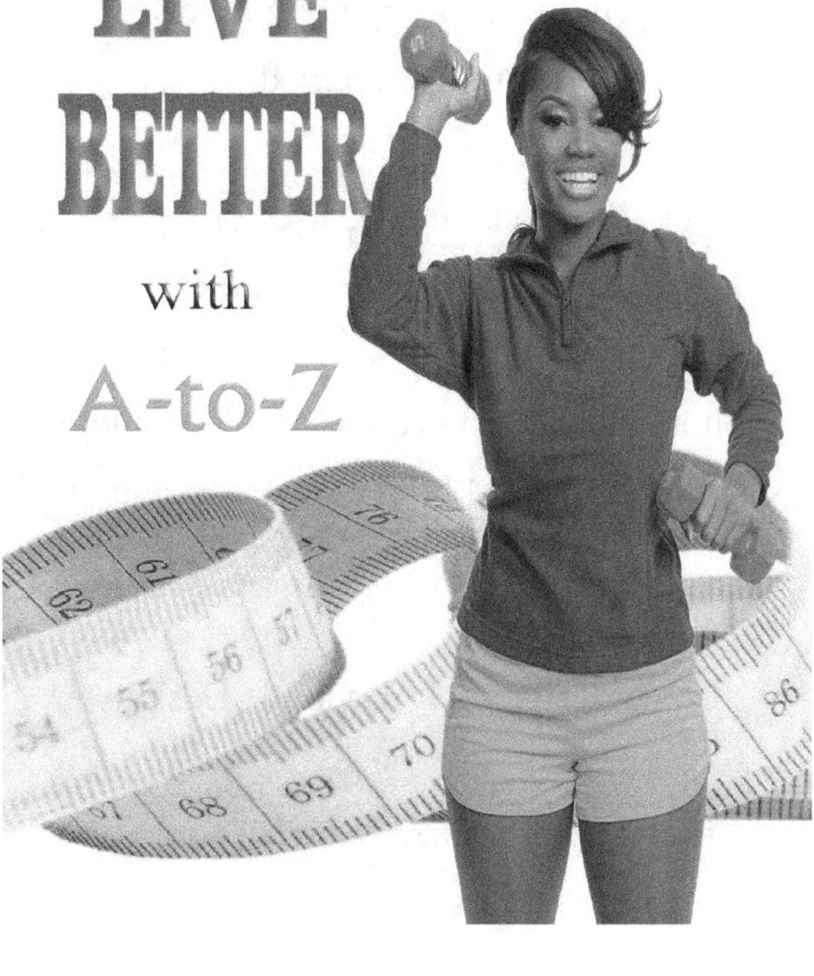

Acknowledgements

I am most grateful to God for giving me the inspiration and desire to share my knowledge with others. I am thankful for the continuous support of my loving parents and their presence in my life. A special thanks is extended to my mother, Ifeoma McNeal, for helping me to bring into fruition my first book. I am also appreciative of my beautiful siblings, family, and friends who have over the years motivated me to become skillful in the areas of fitness, nutrition, and better healthcare.

Table of Contents

About Live Better with A-to-Z

When it comes to living a healthy life and knowing what to do, it can be a bit complicated. Live Better with A-to-Z is intended to simplify readers' efforts to living better and serve as an informative and nutritional guide of what Olivia McNeal believes are essential necessities to include for maximum results for a holistic approach to being fit, balanced, looking good, and feeling good.

Whether you are gaining new insight on a vegetable, fruit, vitamin, herb, or supplement or being reminded of a familiar health strategy that works, this book filled with 26 proven and research-based tips will renew and supercharge you to continue making progress on your healthcare journey to realizing your goals. This is the right quick handy informational guide for you.

Your purchase of this book was another step in the right direction of your commitment to living a better life. It speaks volumes, and I thank you. This quick reference guide of A-to-Z essentials will serve as a supplement booster to help you yield even more positive results.

Insight gained from reading this book and active use of its content will do the following:

1. Promote Weight Loss
2. Improve Focus
3. Improve Life Results
4. Promote Skin Rejuvenation
5. Increase Daily Energy
6. Improve Muscle Recovery
7. Improve Blood Pressure
8. Improve Blood Glucose
9. Improve Joint Inflammation
10. Improve Circulation
11. Improve Cholesterol
12. Counteract Depression
13. Increase Metabolism

Let's get started with Olivia McNeal's Live Better with A-to-Z!

A

Amino Acids

A for Amino acids. Did you know that your body in fact needs more than 20 total amino acids to build and repair muscles and tissues? It's important to know which foods will help you get the right amount of amino acids. Amino acids are the building blocks that join together by peptide bonding to later make proteins. Let's briefly discuss proteins in order to appreciate the micro chemical units called amino acids.

Proteins make up a great part of the body, in fact, it is second-largest component to water in body composition percentage. Proteins make up muscles, joint systems, organs, bone and skeletal systems. Proteins are responsible for important things to us like hair, skin, and athletic ability. Every day protein is being broken down into amino acids, so think of each amino acids as toy blocks joining together to make a bigger product. Each amino acid is different and comes together for a distinct purpose in creating bodily needs. If the body needs it, it will create it and amino acids are the essentials to this process.

If amino acids are in sufficient amounts, then protein synthesis is weakened resulting in metabolism dysfunction and limitations. Young adults and older both need amino acids in sufficient supply to avoid negative effects such as weight problems, hair loss, sleep disorders, diabetes, erectile disorders. Amino acids consumption also improves arthritis, cardiovascular imbalance, and even menopausal complaints.

Common amino acids to look for on nutrition fact labels and a list of foods high in amino acids are included in the box below.

Common Amino Acids	Foods High in Amino Acids
Histidine	Beef
Isoleucine	Pork
Leucine	Poultry and Seafood
Lysine	Turkey
Methionine	Chicken
Phenylalanine	Eggs (Dairy Products)
Threonine	Milk
Tryptophan	Yogurt
Valine	Cheese

B

Berries

B for berries, B for great benefits! Berries are packed with antioxidants with natural fiber, anti-cancer agents, and nutrients that support good memory and a healthy digestive system. Berries are fun to eat.

I know many are concerned about when to buy fresh berries as they can become very costly when purchased "out of season". It's important to know that berries do not have to be purchased or consumed as fresh fruit; berries or berry supplements can be bought in capsules over the counter. There are no excuses when it comes to living a healthy, balanced life! I encourage you to make living better a high priority and have fun doing it.

Common berry favorites are acai berry, blueberries, cranberries, raspberries, and strawberries, and chili peppers. Yes, chili peppers are surprisingly considered a berry. Ask any botanist. The seeds within, by definition, make chili peppers and other fun foods such as avocado, eggplant, okra, and tomatoes technically fruit though they are not known for having a sweet taste.

Strawberry: Strawberries are rich in antioxidant which enables it to neutralize metals in the body that carry more negative charges. Doing this allow strawberries to be great anti-aging benefits. Strawberries boost your metabolism because they are rich with Vitamin C, Magnesium, and Fiber.

Here's a Skin Care Tip: Add strawberries to your classic Apple Cider Vinegar (ACV) and bentonite clay mask. This regimen prepares a better smelling mixture with a more earth tone color.

How to Make a Strawberry + ACV Clay Mask

Prepares 2 facials

1 tablespoon of bentonite clay

2 full strawberries (mashed)

1 teaspoon of ACV

2 teaspoons of water

This Strawberry + ACV clay mask helps reduce acne, clears

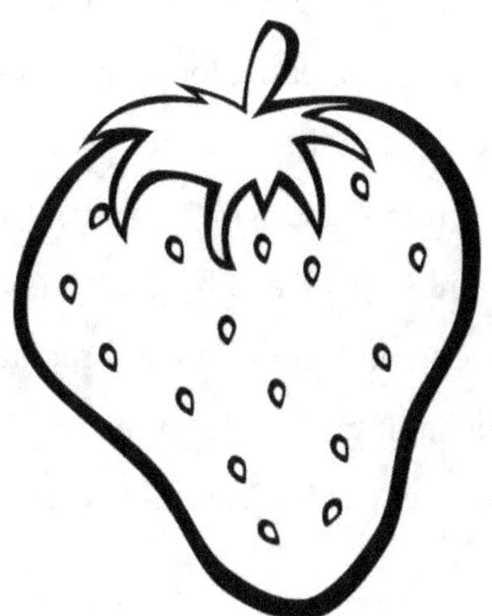

scars, and serves as an anti-aging mask keeping the skin tight and bright. All of the ingredients used to make this mask may be found at a local food market.

Blueberry: Blueberries are rich in Vitamin B6 and Vitamin C and it's a source of potassium and fiber. Adding blueberries to your grocery list regularly can help lower cholesterol which improves overall heart health, reducing your risk of heart attacks and strokes. Blueberries can be used as toppings, incorporated in any baking recipe, and added to a daily snack.

Raspberry: Raspberries are unique because they contain acid that prevents the growth of tumor causing cells. They are also known for containing vitamins, fiber, and antioxidants.

Cranberry: Cranberries are known to improve urinary tract health, decrease blood pressure, immune systems functioning because of the nutrients found in them. Cranberry is a type of supreme food which contains antioxidant benefits. A cup of cranberries are only 25 calories making this a great snack to keep you feeling full and remaining compliant with a caloric managing diet. The cranberry juice that is unsweetened is the best way to increase the benefits of the cranberry.

Unsweetened cranberry juice and water 5-1 ratio. Prepare drink for week and drink 1 glass daily. This will decrease the frequency of colds and infections.

Açaí Berry: Acai berry includes a high level of antioxidant benefits; it's the highest antioxidant strength among fruits.

Small changes can make a huge
difference.

C

Carbohydrates vs. Carbs

Carbohydrates are most commonly called carbs. Carbs are found in most foods and supplements. Carbs over time have gotten a bad reputation because they are found in bread, pasta, and sweets. They also contribute to weight gain, but in fact, carbohydrates are responsible for energy. So, let's not throw carbs out just yet. As you navigate through this guide and become more informed on certain essentials to include in your daily regimen, know that balance is vital with everything.

Carbs fuel the body to do its everyday functions. Functions as big as a four-mile run or an unseen activity like the rebuilding of cells are fueled by carbs. Carbs are partially made of a sugar called saccharides, so the body uses carbs to be broken down into disaccharides or sugars to produce glucose or energy. The body either uses this energy or stores it. It is important to note that all carbs are carbohydrates, but not all carbohydrates are carbs.

Carbohydrates can be quite confusing to understand. Essentially, carbohydrates are divided into two groups-simple carbohydrates and complex carbohydrates.

Simple carbohydrates called simple sugars, include fructose (fruit sugar), sucrose (table sugar), and lactose (milk sugar).

Complex carbohydrates contain sugar too, but the sugar molecules are combined to form complex chains. Complex carbohydrates include fiber and starches. Foods rich in complex carbohydrates are vegetables, whole grains, peas, and beans. Try to eat unrefined carbohydrate foods instead of refined, processed foods such as soft drinks, desserts, candy, and sugar. Avoid foods that are nutrient poor.

About 50 to 60 percent of your total daily calories should come from carbohydrates, much of which should consist of healthy complex carbohydrates to include the right amount of fiber. Much of your fiber intake will come from whole grains, fruits, and vegetables.

D
Detox

Detoxing is helpful to rid the body from toxins, disrobe buildup, and oxidation. Adding antioxidant powerful fruit to water through diffusion can aid in resetting your metabolism. Add fruits to a water-filled container of your choice. Drink 32 fluid ounces daily.

Add fruit such as strawberries, blueberry, and lemons to your water to achieve the maximum benefits. The key to a successful series is to avoid consumption of sugary drinks such as juices and sodas. A 7 day, 14 day, or 30 day detox is vital to cleansing the body and aiding in weight loss and vitality.

E

Enzymes

Enzymes are important because they are proteins that control the speed of chemical reactions in your body. Without enzymes, these reactions would take place too slowly to keep you alive. Some enzymes, like the ones in your gut, break down large molecules into smaller ones. Others, like the enzymes that make DNA, use small molecules to build up large complex ones. Enzymes also help cells to communicate with each other, keeping cell growth, and cell death under control.

The body naturally produces digestive enzyme with your saliva and mucus of the stomach. Together with added enzymes and fiber they help to ensure foods eaten are broken down and bulked to ensure the body is able to rid itself of wasteful materials. Overall, this helps you to achieve total bowel harmony and gut support.

Below is a list of enzymes found in foods and capsules that can be purchased at grocery stores and pharmacies. The next time you're in a grocery store, read the nutrition label for foods found with these enzymes:

Amylase, Bromelain, Cellulase, Chymopapain, Diastase, Glucoamylase, hemicellulase, Hyaluronidase, Invertase, Lactase, lipase, Maltase, Pancreatin, Papin, Pectinase, Pepsin, Phytase, Plasmin, Protease, Renin, Trypsin

A healthy outside starts from the inside.

F

Fiber

Fiber is a dietary material containing substances such as cellulose, lignin, and pectin, which are resistant to the action of digestive enzymes. Fiber, like carbs, are carbohydrates that are broken down; however, unlike carbs, fiber can not break down into simple sugars that lead to fat storage. Yayyy!!!

Fiber on the other hand converts into water or bulk. That is why fiber is important to digestion and regularity, weight management, blood sugar regulation, and cholesterol maintenance. Its ability to maintain shape in the body is unique.

Fiber, in addition with a hydrated balance to the body's digestion system, will strengthen the body and produce overall health and bowel relief. Daily fiber intake should be 25-30 grams. Listed below are foods high in fiber to consume.

Fiber Foods (average grams of fiber per serving)		
Apples 4.4 g	Whole Grain Bread 3 g	Bran Cereal 4.2 g
Berries 3.6 g	Oatmeal 4 g	Vegetables 4g

G

Ginger, Ginseng, Garlic

Ginger, ginseng, and garlic can be incorporated in your diet by cooking with them or consuming capsules with theses active ingredients. Daily consumption of these can reduce belly fat, increase daily energy, and improve cholesterol and blood pressure. Let's discuss each ingredient individually.

13 reasons to include ginger in your diet.

1. Ginger can relieve nausea
2. Ginger can reduce bad cholesterol (LDL)
3. Ginger can promote gut health
4. Ginger can prevent cancer
5. Ginger can relieve pain
6. Ginger contains minerals
7. Ginger relieves muscle soreness
8. Ginger improves memory
9. Ginger reduces blood pressure
10. Ginger relieves menstrual cramps

11. Ginger is an anti-inflammatory

12. Ginger kills bacteria

13. Ginger provides osteoarthritis relief

13 reasons to include ginseng in your diet

1. Ginseng increases energy

2. Ginseng reduces fatigue

3. Ginseng improves cognitive function

4. Ginseng provides lung support

5. Ginseng lowers blood sugar

6. Ginseng is an anti-inflammatory

7. Ginseng improves sexual performance

8. Ginseng aids in weight loss

9. Ginseng boost immune systems

10. Ginseng treats menstrual cramps and menopausal discomfort

11. Ginseng treats ADHD

12. Ginseng relieves stress

13. Ginseng reduces alcohol toxicity

13 reasons to include Garlic in your diet

1. Garlic controls blood pressure

2. Garlic improves immune system

3. Garlic reduces bad cholesterol

4. Garlic prevents Alzheimer's

5. Garlic provides detox benefits

6. Garlic improves postmenopausal bone health

7. Garlic is an antibacterial digestion support

8. Garlic prevents blood clotting

9. Garlic treats yeast infections

10. Garlic reduces asthma exacerbation

11. Garlic improves eye health

12. Garlic promotes liver support

13. Garlic treats eczema

H

Herbs

Did you know that about 80 percent of the world's population uses herbs and plants to treat various common ailments? This proves that the use of herbs is nothing new. Herbalism is often times forgotten in everyday practice. Pharmaceutical companies were originally founded upon the ability to isolate certain active ingredients into the purest form by way of organic chemistry and medicinal medicine techniques. Remember the next time the next you are facing a bodily ailment, herbs can help. Today's medicines have evolved from herbs and still contain herbal supplements as the major ingredient. Herbs in appropriate daily dosing are safer than prescribed medications, however, you should still consult with your doctor and pharmacist about potential drug interactions with current supplements and medications.

Herbs can be found in grocery stores and vitamin shops in the form of capsules, pills, teas, and oils. Listed below are is an alphabetical list of some herbs and their use benefits to familiarize yourself with.

Aloe- Aloe acts as an astringent and antibacterial and heals skins and body sores. Consumed, it helps to lower cholesterol, soothes stomach irritation, aids healing, and acts as a laxative.

Ashwagandha- Ashwagandha helps improve mental sharpness, increases physical endurance, and improves sexual function.

*Bilberry-*Bilberry helps control insulin levels and keeps blood vessels flexible, increasing blood flow.

*Black Walnut-*Black walnut aids digestion, heal throat sores, cleanses the body of parasites, and acts as a laxative.

*Cayenne-*Cayenne aids digestion, weight loss, and stops bleeding ulcers. Cayenne helps to get rid of colds, sinus infections, and sore throats.

*Chamomile-*Chamomile stimulates the appetite, aids digestion and sleep, and reduces stress and anxiety.

*Dandelion-*Dandelion acts as a diuretic, cleanses the blood and liver, and improves functioning of the kidneys and stomach.

Devil's Claw-Devil's claw is great for relieving back pain, migraines, and arthritis.

Echinacea-Echinacea works to heal the immune system and fights cold and flu symptoms.

Eucalyptus-Eucalyptus is a decongestant good for cold relief.

Fenugreek-Fenugreek helps lower cholesterol and blood sugar levels. It also reduces fever, helps with asthma, and is good for the eyes.

Ginkgo-Ginkgo improves brain functioning and aids against depression, dementia, asthma, and kidney disorders.

Green tea-Green tea lower cholesterol levels, protects against cancer, fights tooth decay, combats mental fatigue, and helps regulate insulin levels.

Horse Chestnut-Horse chestnut reduces excess tissue fluids, eases nighttime muscle spasms in the legs, and good for varicose veins.

Irish Moss-Irish Moss is good for bronchitis and intestinal disorders.

Lavender-Lavender relieves stress and depression and is good for psoriasis and other skin problems.

Maca-Maca increases energy and helps with anemia, chronic fatigue, and menopausal symptoms.

Marshmallow-Marshmallow aids the body in getting rid of excess fluid and mucus.

Nettle-Nettle is a pain reliever. It helps relieves arthritis, inflammation, and helps stimulate hair growth.

Olive leaf-Olive leaf helps fight colds, flu, and all types of bacteria, and viruses.

Rhodiola - Rhodiola improves cognitive energy and fights mental and physical fatigue. This herb is ideal for athletes and those who suffer from depression. Rhodiola reduces stress and anxiety, prevents Alzheimer, and enhances sex drive and mood.

St. John's Wort- St. John's Wort helps control stress and overtime improves depression symptoms and can be used with children or adults who have been diagnosed to have Attention Deficit Hyperactivity Disorder (ADHD).

Tea Tree-Tea Tree is used to disinfect wounds and heals acne, athlete's foot, and other skin cuts and breakouts.

Uva Ursi-Uva Ursi fights bacteria and strengthens heart muscle.

Valerian-Valerian improves circulation, lowers blood pressure, and treats insomnia. Valerian can also act as a stress and pain reliever shown to promote better sleep.

White Willow-White Willow is a bark that is good for treating allergies, cramps, and other pains that affect the nerve, joints, and back.

Yohimbe-Yohimbe improves sex drive by increasing blood flow and also increases testosterone levels.

I

Intermittent fasting

Intermittent fasting is a way for the body to better burn fat by way of using foods consumed during feeding cycles to be used as immediate energy. Once that energy is used, the body goes into fasting mode as it is then forced to use stored fat that once was sugar and carbohydrates as energy. Overtime intermittent fasting schedules need to be alternated. You can alternate it by simply changing the fasting scheduled times weekly. This increases caloric burn and tricks the metabolism weekly aiding in an overall better feeling helping keep fasting up.

 A fasting schedule is first made by deciding which 16 hours your body will be fasting and the 8-hour window you will be feeding. The most popular intermittent fasting is the 18/6 ratio, where you eat twice from 10 am -6 pm or 12p- 8pm and this is known as your feeding window. Be sure to eat twice in one window, not both. It is ideal to eat twice during your window incorporating protein, fiber, minerals, vitamins, and color rich food items on the menu. This helps you remain consistent with your fasting and see results without breaking the fast inappropriately. You also can limit your meals to once a day improving results but also emphasizes the importance of consuming the body's daily need in only one meal. Be sure to consult with your doctor and pharmacist for your safe and healthy daily calorie quantity. This is decided based on physical activity, gender, height, and weight.

Fasting windows during intermittent fasting can be a schedule that fits your daily activities like work, exercise, cooking, and cleaning. It is important to pick a window that is in alignment with your goals. For instance, if your goal is to lose body fat you should consider skipping evening meals and making your feeding window earlier in the day, resulting in better digestive tract functioning at night and forcing the body to use stored fat to accomplish evening duties. Be sure to break the fast with breakfast to speed metabolism and resupply the body with nutrients for the day ahead.

J

Juices and liquid calories

When most think of calories, they think of calories in solids and foods. Many forget to monitor the calorie intake from juices. Think liquid calories. Liquid calories are liquid phase drinks that contain calories from carbs, sugar, protein, or other ingredients. This means that you can consume calories through juices, smoothies, or blended mixtures.

A calorie is a word that describes the amount of energy needed. So food calories describe the amount of energy or burn needed to breakdown the particular food items. A caloric burn is the amount of energy use. Therefore, if you can count the amount of calories consumed each day you can calculate the amount of activity need to burn. This puts you in control of your body. Begin to count the calories added in each ingredient added to take better control of your body.

Juices that are not high in sugar can relieve the digestive tract of its daily duty and allows even it to rest and reset. This in turn improves abdominal appearance and regularity. Juices are indeed liquid calories and should be viewed as such. Just remember not all liquid calories are juice.

It's never too early or too late to work toward being the healthiest you.

K

Know your limitations

Know Your Limitations and expect your weakness. This in turn will make you stronger.

Learning and understanding the factors that stand in your way of better health is one of the keys to achieving goals. Ever heard the saying minor setback for a major comeback? This means you must fail a few times to learn what works and what doesn't. Other nutritionist and fitness professionals can help advise and educate you, but personal effort is needed to be involved in your own process. The emphasis is understanding the behavior, naming the behavior so that you can unlearn the behavior and through conditioning replace the behavior with a more productive and more beneficial one. This allows you to begin to identify certain thoughts, routines, that hinders growth and make an effort to replace this or improve performance with more planning and positive thinking.

L

Lemons

Lemons are rich in Vitamin C, Fiber, and contain a great source of citric acid. These key components of the lemon allow it to improve the immune system, boost metabolism, decrease bad cholesterol (LDL), and brighten skin. Lemons improve acne and possess healing qualities that help the body eliminate waste easier and improve blemishes overtime. It also has anti-aging benefits.

The skin facial recipe below will remove dark spots, improve wrinkles, and promote new skin growth.

Lemon Face Mask

1 teaspoon of freshly squeezed lemon juice

1 teaspoon of honey

Oily Skin: add 1 completely mashed fruit or 1 egg

Dry Skin: Add 1 tablespoon of yogurt

M
Minerals

Minerals such as Boron, Calcium, Copper, Iodine, Magnesium, Manganese, Phosphorus, Silicon, Sodium, Zinc play a vital role in chemical processes. The body oftentimes needs more of a certain kind of ingredient to perform a certain action. If the body is lacking in that ingredient, it will cause delayed responses and results.

Although foods and vegetables are often rich in these minerals they can also be found in a multivitamin. Multivitamin should be taken with water and a meal to prevent gastric intestinal irritation.

N

Nutrition Facts

Watch what you eat! I can't stress enough the importance of clearly understanding how to read and interpret nutrition facts labels.

A nutrition label is used so manufacturing companies can get a product approved by the United States Food and Drug Administration (FDA) and also to inform consumers of the contents inside. Nutrition labels display the serving size, serving per container, calorie count per serving, calories from fat per serving, mineral, protein, cholesterol, sodium (salt), mineral, vitamin, and percentage of other ingredients included. Most nutrition labels are based on a 2,000 or 2,500 daily calorie diet and the values can increase or decrease based on individual calorie need and use.

To avoid being fooled keep in mind that all value percentages are the consumption for each serving size.

*Pay attention to the total fat, cholesterol, and sodium information section. Total fat, saturated fat, and sodium are all bad for your health; limit these nutrients. You want to select foods extremely low in fats and sodium and high percentages in vitamins and minerals.

A serving size shows you all the nutrition quantities per that one serving not the entire container. A serving per container is usually a number that allows you to see how many servings is in one container. Common units used are milligrams and there are 1,000 milligrams in one grams be aware of this if you are counting the daily contents consumed.

A sample nutrition label

Nutrition Facts
Serving Size
Servings Per Container

Amount Per Serving

Calories   Calories from Fat

% Daily Value*

Total Fat
    Saturated Fat
    Trans Fat
Cholesterol
Sodium
Total Carbohydrate
    Dietary Fiber
    Sugars
Protein

Vitamin

*Percent Daily Values are based on a 2,000 calorie diet.

O
Oils

Usually oils don't come to mind first when people think of health. Oils have amazing health benefits and support natural healing. Using oils to improve health were used in ancient days more than 3,000 year ago for cooking and making scents and herbal healing remedies.

Oils are fats that are broken down into saturated or trans fatty acids which are bad for you. Monounsaturated and polyunsaturated fats, though, are heart-healthy alternatives.

Oils can be purchased as liquids or pill supplements.

Names of some essential, good oils are listed below.

Omega-3 Primrose oil	Olive oil
Salmon oil	Black seed oil
Flaxseed oil	Emu oil
MCT oil	Grapeseed oil

P

Protein

Proteins are made up of various combinations of amino acids. They regulate the body's water balance and maintain the proper internal pH. Making protein 30 percent of calories consumed daily can optimize weight loss. Ideally, 150 grams of protein would be appropriate for a person on a 2000- calorie diet. The average man that is not active should consume 56 grams per day and the average inactive woman should consume 46 grams per day of protein. Essentially, the more active a person is the more protein rich diet the person should have. Protein deficiency can upset the body's fluid balance causing edema. Edema is when excess fluid is retained generally around the lower limbs and causing weight gain. Proteins can be found in eggs, meats, and hummus. Protein is commonly found in whey supplements that form flavored or unflavored drinks.

Q

Quinoa

Quinoa is a gluten-free carbohydrate that is sure to fuel your body. It is an easy replacement for rice and other carbohydrates that don't provide such benefits.

Quinoa contains 64 grams of carbohydrates and of that 7 grams of fiber. Quinoa also contains vitamin A, B1, B2, B3, B6, B9, choline, Vitamin C , Vitamin E, Calcium, iron, Magnesium, manganese, phosphorus, potassium, sodium, and zinc. Quinoa has 13.3 grams of water, 14.1 grams of protein, and only 6 grams of fats in every 100 grams of uncooked quinoa.

Using 2 cups of water for every 1 cup of quinoa cook for 10 to 15 minutes until quinoa is tender and water has been absorbed. Add this to any meal to serve as daily carb consumption.

R

Reset

A Reset can be a switch up from your basic actions to thinking of better ways to make solutions. Reset can be just what you need to discontinue poor behaviors, so don't forget to reset your body, way of thinking, and exercise overtime. It's good to switch things up and allow your body to be challenged. Take a moment to notice the things you are doing that are not good practice. Just think to yourself the most common meals you've consumed over the last 2 weeks.

Take a few moments and allow your memory to take your lifestyle into consideration and reflect on your sleep, morning routine, and the number of time you engage in physical activity. All these things play a vital role in metabolism, which in turn determines your well-being. Make plans to do better by incorporating more healthy habits into your life, such as improve sleep, eating habits, oils that you cook with and more.

It won't be perfect, because nothing is; but do your best to improve. This will in turn motivate you to achieve more and more in your health journey or inspire you to always reset.

Nothing looks as good as healthy feels.

S

Sodium and salt

According to research, 1500 milligrams of sodium each day is a sodium intake goal you should consider adopting that is ideal. When you grocery shop and view nutrition labels, you may notice that sodium is in nearly every food item. This is mainly because of sodium's ability to enhance flavor and preserve food.

On average, one person consumes about 3,400 milligrams of salt, mostly deriving from processed and canned foods. This is not good.

Sodium aids in electrolyte balance, water balance, and the body cannot function without sodium. With this said, it is important to consume sodium in moderation though as high salt diets leads to high blood pressure and heart disease.

Did you know that 40% of salt's weight is sodium? When you consume salt, you are getting more than double the amount of salt than sodium. Try to consume unrefined varieties of salt, like sea salt. There is no need to obsessively count the milligram of sodium but simply:

1. Add a small amount of salt when appropriate for taste at the end of preparation for better taste.

2. Eat real, fresh food and avoid or reduce the amount of frozen, canned, and processed food consumed.

3. Read nutrition labels before every purchase to ensure you are not consumed too much sodium. Remember 1500 milligrams or less of sodium consumption daily is ideal.

T

Turmeric

Have you ever heard of turmeric? On cooking shows, chefs pronounce it "TOO-mer-ic". Turmeric is an anti-inflammatory natural herb and very strong antioxidant. You can find this natural herb easily at vitamin shops, grocery stores, and online sites. Turmeric looks like grounded cinnamon and can also be found in liquid or pill form.

The benefits of turmeric are almost endless and the demand for this spice has become popular in the marketplace over years as more people realize its many uses. Turmeric is used to help prevent cancer, heal acne as an antibacterial, heal wounds faster, reduce inflammation, lower high blood pressure, reduce stress, relieve cramps and arthritis as a natural pain reliever, and lighten and tighten skin just to list a few of the health benefits of turmeric.

As a brief testimonial, I once took two capsules of turmeric by mouth to alleviate pain I was experiencing in my right hand thumb. I felt relief within 20 minutes.

A recommended daily dose of tumeric is 300 milligram. For safety purposes, do not exceed 1,000 milligrams a day.

If you are dealing with insomnia and have difficulty falling asleep, consider preparing and drinking a cup of Turmeric Milk to help induce for you a good sleep.

How to Make Turmeric Milk

First, add ¾ teaspoon of Turmeric to a cup of boiled milk. Second, stir the mixture and let it cool until it is at a desired warm temperature. Third, drink it. Diabetics should not add sugar.

Turmeric Face Masks

The best acne-fighting face masks to use are ones made with turmeric. Turmeric removes bacteria, lightens skins, fades acne pores, tightens skins, and reduces dark circles. Don't be alarmed by its yellow or orange mask color. It works!

A few drops of squeezed, fresh Lemon Juice + ½ teaspoon of Turmeric Powder + 1 Egg white = a nice turmeric face mask.

U

You

Yep, you guessed it U is for Y-O-U. The key to living better is you. It is all about the choices you make, so let's make better ones each day. It is important to take care of yourself in all aspects and truly understand your unique abilities. This in turn improves self-image, self-esteem, and self-love. Often people are blocked mentally or don't understand the body they live in and begin to get frustrated with the health journey. Let's not get frustrated but instead always remember that you get what you put in, so your health reflects your daily habits. The first step is to learn which body type you have. There are three different types: ectomorphs, endomorphs, and mesomorphs. This is important because once you determine your body type you must then create a realistic goal. Often times people want to achieve a physique that simply too challenging of a transformation based on the body type they have. People also develop poor habits that simply work against achieving their goals. Let's discuss.

Ectomorphs are those naturally lean and long and have difficulty building muscle. Endomorph are those who have high body fat percentages and have pear shaped figures.

Endomorphs are proven to storing more fat than the other two types.

Mesomorphs are those whom are naturally muscular and have high metabolisms helping them convert consumed substances into energy quickly and protein into muscle easily. Goal setting is the next step after you determine which body type you possess. Below are examples of goals for each body type and things that will help achieve them.

For my Ectomorphs:

Your Goal might be to gain muscle and weight.

My Advice: Ectomorphs tend to burn calories fast so to achieve these results add carbohydrate and protein rich items to your meals as toppings, like peanut butter (high in protein and sugar), avocado (high in fat), seeds (high in fiber and protein) and yogurt (high in fat). Snack at least 3 times a day with at least 150 calories in each snack.

For my Endomorphs:

A Common Goal is to Lose inches and weight.

Advice: Endomorphs tend to hold on to fats more readily, so the action plan is to burn more calories than is consumed to lose inches and weight. Activity should be at least 15 minutes of cardio daily this helps with consistent metabolism boosting. It is also vital to break the fast with a caloric smart breakfast including fiber, fruits, vegetables, and protein followed by a light workout to get the body started with burning calories throughout the day ahead. Intentionally cut back on sugars and simple carbs. Do high intensity exercise meaning it should be hard to talk or sing for about 30 minutes 3-4 days a week.

For my Mesomorphs

The Goal might be to gain curves or get lean.

Advice: Consume a healthy fat rich diet (olive oil, coconut oil, and avocado) with high intensity cardio of about 30 minutes 3-4 days a week to get lean or strength train for 60 minutes 3-4 day a week to gain curves.

V
Vitamins

Vitamins are vital substances for cell function, growth, and development. We will discuss the 13 essential vitamins that aid in proper functionality. A vitamin deficiency can cause unwanted health issues. Most whole grains, fruits and vegetables contain certain vitamins and not eating enough can put you at risk for heart disease and cancer to name a few.

Vitamins are divided into two categories, water soluble and fat soluble. Vitamin B1, B2, B3, B5, B6,B7, B9, and B12 are used rapidly because they are water soluble. The parts that are not used or absorbed is eliminated in the urine. Vitamin A, D,E, and K are fat soluble and thus they better absorbed if taken with dairy and fats.

- Vitamin A helps maintain bone and skin health
- Vitamin C is also called ascorbic acid and promotes healthy gums and strong immune system fighting infections and healing wounds.

- Vitamin D helps the body absorb calcium which aids in bone development. You can receive the body's required Vitamin C amount by receiving sunlight for 15 minutes a day.
- Vitamin E aids in Vitamin K absorption and helps produce red blood cells.
- Vitamin K helps blood clot to prevent the body from bleeding out during injury.
- Vitamin B1 is also called thiamine aids in the conversion of carbohydrates into energy for the body to use.
- Vitamin B2 is also called riboflavin is essential for cell growth.
- Vitamin B3 is also called niacin and it improves cholesterol at high doses and at low doses improves skin and nerve health.
- Vitamin B5 is also called pantothenic acid is essential for the metabolism or breakdown of food.
- Vitamin B7 is also called biotin which is needed for protein and carbohydrate metabolism. Biotin also promotes hormone and cholesterol production.
- Vitamin B6 is also called pyridoxine and it helps maintain brain and red blood cell health. The more protein you eat the more Vitamin B6 is needed to maintain protein involved chemical reactions.

- Vitamin B12 is also called cyanocobalamin and is required to maintain metabolism and nervous system health.
- Vitamin B9 is also called Folate or folic acid. Vitamin B9 is needed for DNA synthesis and tissue growth.

Being healthy and fit isn't a fad or a trend. It's a lifestyle.

W
Water

By now you should know the importance of water: its natural healing agents, and many of its benefits. Still, I find that many struggle to consume the amount of water each day that they truly need. This is a serious matter.

Water is about 70 % of our body composition this amount varies from person to person depending on height, weight, physical activity and gender. Daily intake needs vary by these same factors and, on average, an adult should consume 8 glasses of water a day. Water consumption is responsible for digestion, circulation, and excretion. Water helps transport nutrients throughout the body and carries wasteful materials out through processes like sweat and tears. The quality of water has evolved overtime which has led to an increased life spans and protected us from infection and disease. A simple glass of water can alleviate things as anxiety, headache, and other pains.

Tap Water- Improve your tap water by heating it for 3-5 minutes to kill bacteria and parasites. Refrigerated tap water in an uncovered pitcher can improve taste.

Bottled water- Bottled water is sealed and contains some antimicrobial agent that kills parasites and microbes that eventually make its way into the water from household tap streams or flows. The point is bottled water is not much safer than tap water so consider saving money or recycling water bottled to remain hydrated.

Alkaline Water- Alkaline water has a pH higher or more basic than that of the body. This allows the water to neutralize the acid in your body improving reflux, upset stomach, and skin.

Sparkling Water is a healthy soda and alcoholic beverage alternative providing you with the fizz that you crave. Typically on these products, look for "carbonated water" on the nutritional facts label. This indicates that water is the source of the bubbly drink and not other unsafe carbonation forms. Aim for a zero calorie beverage.

Watermelon is a great way to "eat water". It contains 92% water and 6% sugar.

For a nutritious water drink, check out this "Watermelon Sparkly" recipe (prepares approximately 10 cups).

<u>Watermelon Sparkly Drink</u>

1 ½ cup of squeezed lemon juice

4 cups of watermelon juice (serves as sweetener)

2 liters of sparkling water

1 bag of pebble ice

1 pitcher container

X

eXercise

Exercise is the engagement of physical activity that promotes caloric burn, improves mood, and improves stamina. It is time to make physical activity fun and convenient.

Get moving for at least 30 minutes a day most days of the week for a healthy weight loss of about 1-2 pounds a week, if you decrease caloric intake by 250-500 calories daily (also depends on the quality of food consumed). Movement can be done anywhere and yes I said anywhere: office desk, couch, bed, and even the bathtub. Movement to the body improves the immune system, helping the body fight off infections and diseases. Movement also improves flexibility, preventing injury and relieving stress on joints. Movement improves blood circulation which lowers blood pressure and increases sex drive.

Y

Yoga and Meditation

Meditation is known to be a source of inner peace and some still believe it provides healing benefits as well. Here's what I know. Meditation is free. It provides mental space that allows me to feel happier, more balanced, and better rested. Meditation is achieved by breathing, performing body position, and allowing total free fall of your body by remaining planting into the earth continuously. Meditation is often the warm up, continuous effort, and the conclusion to a yoga session.

Yoga can be done in a classroom setting as well but would require access to a community gym or in the comfort of your home. Yoga can be a recreational activity you can enjoy with friends, family and community. Social yoga is a great way to relieve stress, gain core and cardiovascular exercise, and improve blood flow while meeting new people and increasing activity to your life.

Meditation can be achieved by increasing your musical enjoyment, adding more genres to your music collection and taking a moment to breathe and clear your mind.

Meditation can also be a way to enjoy silence. Maybe you hear too many people talking and want to hear your own thoughts. This can be achieved as well.

A peaceful heart leads to a healthy body. What's just as important as getting your body in shape is getting your mind in shape.

Z

Zzz- Sleep

Oh my, the benefits of something as simple as sleeping are insurmountable. The demands of life, daily list of long To Do items, and constant social interaction interfere with the body's need to sleep, rest, and rejuvenate.

You should receive 6-8 hours of sleep every night. This helps with the body's recovery process. During sleep the body digests food, muscles recover from the day's activity, and the brain recovers from its activity and improves memory. Overtime sleep deprivation can impact health in many ways interfering with over rejuvenation making you feel groggy and perform poorly.

If you struggle with going to sleep, night exercise and meditation might be the thing for you. It's important to relax and prepare the body for rest while letting go of worries from the past and the anxiety produced by expecting future events. Without sleep your body isn't able to recharge and make the next day better.

<u>In Conclusion</u>

Readers, I applaud you on your journey to live a better life. I charge you to from this day forward begin intentionally being mindful of your daily consumptions. Hopefully, after reading the Live Better with A-to-Z guide, you are better informed of foods that will support your healthcare efforts and have become more knowledgeable of foods to avoid.

Remember, the goal is to strive for balance. I want you to become more conscientious about what you are putting in your body. Begin to incorporate the A-to-Z essentials into your diet and make a commitment to live better. I'm eager to hear about your results. May the rest of your life be the best of your life.

Contact information

Readers, be sure to follow me on social media and join the live better team. Email me. I am always open to hear from my readers to provide responses, advice, and more tips.

IG: @drlivebetter

Facebook: Olivia D. McNeal

Email: oliviadmcneal@gmail.com